The Art of Happy Living

SIMPLE PLEASURES AND CREATIVE PURSUITS

EVANNIE ROSE

The Art of Happy Living

SIMPLE PLEASURES AND CREATIVE PURSUITS

EVANNIE ROSE

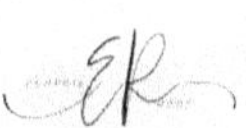

"May your life be filled with simple joys and creative wonders, guiding you on a journey of happiness and fulfillment."
Evannie Rose

Contents

CHAPTER 1

Embracing Mindfulness and Gratitude

"Mindfulness is a way of befriending ourselves and our experience." - Jon Kabat-Zinn.

The Power of Mindfulness

Understand the concept of mindfulness and its benefits.

• Mindfulness is being fully present and engaged at the moment without judgment or distraction. It involves paying attention to our thoughts, feelings, bodily sensations, and environment with openness and curiosity.

• Mindfulness has benefits that include reduced stress and anxiety, improved emotional regulation, enhanced focus and concentration, and increased self-awareness. It can also lead to greater well-being and more profound happiness.

• Mindfulness can be cultivated through various practices, including meditation, deep breathing, and mindful movement. It is a skill that can be developed over time, leading to lasting positive changes in the mind and body.

Learn simple mindfulness exercises for daily practice.

• Mindful Breathing: Sit or lie down in a comfortable position. Close your eyes and bring your attention to your breath. Notice the sensation of the air entering and leaving your nostrils or the rise and fall of your chest or abdomen. When your mind wanders, gently bring your focus back to your breath. Practice this for 5-10 minutes daily.

• Body Scan Meditation: Begin by lying down or sitting comfortably. Close your eyes and start by focusing on the sensations in your feet. Gradually move your attention through each body part, noticing tension, warmth, or other sensations. This exercise helps you become more attuned to your body's needs and promotes relaxation.

• Mindful Walking: Choose a quiet place to walk indoors or outdoors. As you walk, pay attention to your body's movement and the sensation of your feet touching the ground. Observe your surroundings, noting the colors, sounds, and smells. This practice helps integrate mindfulness into everyday activities.

Explore how mindfulness can enhance appreciation for life's moments.

• Practicing mindfulness allows us to slow down and savor the richness of life's experiences. By being fully present, we can appreciate the beauty in simple moments, whether it's the warmth of the sun on our skin, the taste of a delicious meal, or the laughter of a loved one.

• Mindfulness helps us develop a sense of gratitude for the present moment, which can lead to greater happiness and fulfillment. It encourages us to let go of worries about the past or future and embrace the joy available to us right now.

• By cultivating mindfulness, we can deepen our connection to ourselves and the world around us, leading to a more meaningful and contented life.

Cultivating Gratitude

We are discovering the positive impacts of gratitude on happiness.

• Gratitude is the practice of recognizing and appreciating the positive aspects of life. It has been shown to significantly impact happiness and well-being by shifting focus from what is lacking to what is abundant.

• Studies have found that individuals who regularly practice gratitude experience increased joy, optimism, and life satisfaction. They also tend to have stronger relationships, better physical health and reduced stress and depression.

• Gratitude fosters a positive mindset, helping individuals to cope with adversity, savor positive experiences, and build resilience. It can create a virtuous cycle where gratitude leads to happiness, which fosters more gratitude.

Practice gratitude through journaling and reflection.

• Gratitude Journaling: One of the most effective ways to cultivate gratitude is by keeping a gratitude journal. Daily, write down three to five things you are grateful for. These can be big or small, from a beautiful sunset to a kind gesture from a friend. This practice helps train the mind to notice and appreciate the positive aspects of life.

• Reflection: Set aside time each week to reflect on your gratitude journal entries. Consider the impact these positive experiences have had on your life. This reflection can deepen your sense of appreciation and enhance your overall sense of well-being.

• Sharing Gratitude: Share your gratitude with others. Expressing appreciation to friends, family, or colleagues strengthens your relationships and amplifies gratitude's positive effects on your happiness.

Incorporate gratitude rituals into your daily routine.

• Morning Gratitude: Start your day with a gratitude ritual. Before getting out of bed, take a few moments to think about what you are grateful for. This sets a positive tone for the day ahead.

• Gratitude Reminders: Place visual reminders around your home or workspace to prompt you to reflect on gratitude throughout the day. This could be a quote, a photograph, or a simple note.

• Evening Reflection: End your day with gratitude. Before going to sleep, remember your day and identify moments or experiences you are grateful for. This can help you end the day on a positive note and improve the quality of your sleep.

You can enhance your happiness and create a more fulfilling life by consciously cultivating gratitude. Gratitude is not just a feeling; it's a practice that requires intention and effort, but the rewards are profound and lasting.

Mindful Eating and Cooking

Experience the joy of mindful eating and savoring flavors.

• Mindful eating is the practice of paying full attention to the experience of eating and drinking, both inside and outside the body. It involves noticing the colors, smells, textures, and flavors of food and the thoughts and feelings that arise while eating.

• To practice mindful eating, take small bites, chew slowly, and savor each mouthful. Notice the different flavors and textures, and appreciate the nourishment the food provides. This practice can enhance the enjoyment of food, reduce overeating, and improve digestion.

• Mindful eating also involves being aware of hunger and fullness cues, eating without distraction, and recognizing the emotional and psychological factors that influence eating habits. By eating mindfully, you can develop a healthier relationship with food and enjoy the pleasures of eating more fully.

Find pleasure in cooking as a form of mindfulness.

• Cooking can be a meditative and enjoyable activity when approached mindfully. It offers an opportunity to be creative, engage the senses, and connect with the present moment.

• To practice mindfulness while cooking, focus on the process rather than the outcome. Pay attention to the colors of the ingredients, the sounds of chopping and sizzling, and the aromas that fill the kitchen. Allow yourself to be fully immersed in the experience.

• Cooking can be a time to slow down and unwind. Enjoy the tactile sensations of handling ingredients and the satisfaction of creating something nourishing and delicious. Cooking mindfully can transform it from a chore into a joyful and relaxing activity.

Create a gratitude list for the food on your table.

• Take a moment before each meal to reflect on the food journey to your table. Consider the farmers who grew the ingredients, the transport that brought them to your store, and the effort you put into preparing the meal.

• Create a gratitude list for the food you eat, acknowledging the abundance and variety available to you. This can include the nutritious value of the food, the pleasure it brings to your taste buds and the cultural or personal significance it holds.

• Expressing gratitude for your food can deepen your appreciation for the interconnectedness of life and the earth's bounty. It can also inspire more conscious and sustainable food choices, contributing to a healthier planet and a more fulfilled you.

Nature Walks and Outdoor Activities

You are engaging in mindful walks to connect with nature.

• Mindful walking involves being fully aware of each step and the environment around you. It is a simple yet powerful way to connect with nature and cultivate mindfulness.

• Choose a natural setting for your walk, such as a park, forest, or beach. As you walk, focus on the sensation of your feet touching the ground, the rhythm of your breath, and the sounds and sights of nature around you.

• Allow yourself to be fully present in the moment, letting go of any distracting thoughts or worries. Observe the details of the natural world, such as the patterns of leaves, the colors of the sky, and the movement of wildlife. This practice can help you feel grounded, calm, and connected to the earth.

Practice gratitude for the beauty of the natural world.

• Take time during your walks or outdoor activities to express gratitude for nature's beauty and abundance. Acknowledge the air that fills your lungs, the sun that warms your skin, and the earth that supports your steps.

• Reflect on the intricate web of life and the interconnectedness of all living things. Gratitude for nature can deepen your appreciation for the planet and inspire a sense of stewardship and responsibility for its care.

• Incorporate gratitude into your outdoor activities by pausing to appreciate the natural wonders you encounter, whether a breathtaking view, a vibrant flower, or a serene river.

Explore outdoor activities that promote mindfulness and appreciation.

• Engage in outdoor activities encouraging mindfulness and a deeper connection with nature. This could include gardening, birdwatching, hiking, or sitting quietly in a natural setting.

• Use these activities as opportunities to practice being fully present, observing the details of the natural world, and savoring the experience without distraction.

• Consider incorporating mindful photography into your outdoor adventures. Capture images of nature with intention and attention, focusing on the beauty and uniqueness of each moment. This can help you see the world with fresh eyes and cultivate a deeper appreciation for the natural environment.

By incorporating mindful walks and outdoor activities into your life, you can enhance your connection to nature, promote well-being, and foster a sense of gratitude for the beauty and wonder of the natural world.

Mindful Relationships

Cultivate mindful listening and communication in relationships.

• Mindful listening involves being fully present and attentive when someone is speaking, without interrupting or preparing your response while they are still talking. This allows for deeper understanding and connection.

• Practice active listening by making eye contact, nodding, and reflecting on what you've heard to ensure you understand correctly. This shows the speaker that you value their thoughts and feelings.

• Mindful communication also involves being aware of your emotions and thoughts when interacting with others. Express yourself honestly and kindly, and be open to feedback without becoming defensive.

Express gratitude towards loved ones regularly.

• Regularly expressing gratitude to your loved ones can strengthen your relationships and increase mutual feelings of appreciation and happiness.

• Make it a habit to verbally express your thanks for specific actions or qualities you appreciate in your partner, family, or friends. This can be as simple as saying, "Thank you for making dinner," or "I appreciate your support."

• Write notes of appreciation, send thoughtful messages, or give small tokens of gratitude to show your loved ones how much they mean to you. These gestures can have a lasting impact on the health and happiness of your relationships.

Strengthen bonds through shared mindful experiences.

• Engaging in shared mindful experiences can deepen your connections with others and create meaningful memories. This could include activities like meditating together, taking a mindful walk, or sharing a silent meal where you focus on the experience of eating without conversation.

• Plan regular activities that encourage mindfulness and presence, such as attending a yoga class together, participating in a mindfulness retreat, or simply sitting quietly in nature.

• Use these shared experiences to practice empathy, understanding, and compassion. By being fully present with each other, you can cultivate a more profound sense of connection and intimacy in your relationships.

Incorporating mindfulness into your relationships can enhance communication, allow you to express gratitude more freely, and strengthen the bonds you share with your loved ones.

CHAPTER 2

Discovering Joy in Creative Expression

"Creativity is intelligence having fun." - Albert Einstein.

Artistic Pursuits

Exploring different forms of art as a means of self-expression.

• Art is a powerful medium for expressing thoughts, emotions, and experiences. Explore various art forms, such as painting, drawing, sculpture, photography, or mixed media, to find the one that resonates with you.

• Engage in artistic activities that allow you to express your creativity freely. Experiment with different techniques, materials, and styles to discover what best captures your unique voice.

• Remember that art is a personal journey. It's not about creating perfect pieces but about expressing yourself authentically. Use art to explore your inner world and communicate your perspectives and feelings.

Encourage the creation of art without judgment or expectation.

• Approach your artistic endeavors with an open mind and a non-judgmental attitude. Let go of the need for your art to meet specific standards or expectations. The value of art lies in the process of creation, not just the final product.

• Create a safe and supportive space for yourself and others to engage in art. Encourage experimentation and risk-taking without fear of failure or criticism.

• Practice self-compassion and kindness as you

explore your artistic abilities. Celebrate your efforts and progress, no matter how small, and recognize that every piece of art reflects your unique journey.

Share your art with others to spread happiness.

• Sharing your art can be a joyful and fulfilling experience. It allows you to connect with others, inspire creativity, and spread happiness through your creations.

• Consider displaying your art in your home, giving it as gifts to friends and family, or participating in local art exhibitions or online platforms. Sharing your art can also open up opportunities for feedback and collaboration, enriching your artistic journey.

• Use your art to spread positive messages, uplift spirits, and create community. Art can bring people together and foster a shared appreciation for beauty and creativity.

By embracing artistic pursuits, you can discover a meaningful avenue for self-expression, personal growth, and connection with others. Let your art be a source of joy, inspiration, and happiness in your life and those around you.

Writing for Pleasure

Experience the cathartic effect of writing.

• Writing can be a powerful tool for emotional release and self-discovery. It allows you to articulate thoughts and feelings that might be difficult to express verbally, providing a sense of catharsis and clarity.

• Engage in free writing exercises, where you write continuously without worrying about grammar, punctuation, or structure. This can help you tap into your subconscious and deeply explore your emotions and experiences.

• Use writing to process and make sense of life's challenges and joys. By putting your thoughts on paper, you can gain new perspectives and find solace in self-expression.

Start a personal journal or blog to express your thoughts.

• Keeping a personal journal is a beautiful way to document your daily experiences, reflections, and aspirations. It can serve as a private space for self-expression and personal growth.

• If you're comfortable sharing your thoughts with a broader audience, consider starting a blog. This can be a platform for you to connect with others who share similar interests or experiences and receive community support and encouragement.

• Regularly writing in a journal or blog can help you develop a habit of reflection and mindfulness. It can also enhance your writing skills and provide a sense of accomplishment as you reflect on your entries over time.

Write letters of appreciation to bring joy to others.

• Writing letters of appreciation is a heartfelt way to express gratitude and spread happiness. Take the time to write personalized notes to friends, family, or strangers, acknowledging their kindness, support, or impact on your life.

• In an age of digital communication, receiving a handwritten letter can be a special and meaningful experience. It shows the recipient that you've taken the time and effort to express your gratitude tangibly.

• Writing appreciation letters can also boost one's happiness. Reflecting on the positive aspects of one's relationships and expressing gratitude can enhance one's sense of well-being and strengthen one's connections with others.

Writing for pleasure, whether through journaling, blogging, or crafting letters, offers a range of emotional and social benefits. It can be a source of joy, healing, and connection in your life.

Music and Dance

Discover the emotional uplift of listening to or playing music.

• Music has a profound ability to evoke emotions and uplift the spirit. Whether listening to your favorite songs or playing an instrument, music can provide comfort, joy, and inspiration.

• Experiment with different genres and styles of music to find what resonates with you. Each type of music can offer a unique emotional experience, from the calming sounds of classical music to the energizing beats of rock or pop.

• Playing an instrument can be rewarding for expressing yourself and improving your mood. Whether you're a beginner or an experienced musician, making music can be a form of meditation and a source of personal fulfillment.

Engage in dancing as a form of joyful movement.

• Dancing is a fun way to exercise and a powerful means of expressing emotions and releasing stress. It allows you to connect with your body and the rhythm of the music in a joyful and liberating way.

• You don't need to be a professional dancer to enjoy the benefits of dance. Simply moving to the music in your way can boost your mood and energy levels.

• Consider taking a dance class or joining a dance group to learn new styles, meet new people, and add a social element to your dancing experience.

Create playlists or attend concerts to enhance your musical experience.

• Curate playlists for different moods or activities, such as a relaxing playlist for unwinding after a long day or an upbeat playlist for energizing your workouts.

• Attending live music events, such as concerts or music festivals, can be an exhilarating experience. The energy of live performances and the shared enjoyment with others can amplify the emotional impact of music.

• Sharing music with friends or family can also enhance your experience. Exchange playlists, recommend new artists, or enjoy listening to music together to deepen your connections and create shared memories.

Crafting and DIY Projects

Explore the satisfaction of creating handmade items.

• Crafting and DIY projects offer a hands-on way to express creativity and create something unique. Whether it's knitting, woodworking, pottery, or any other craft, the process of making something by hand can be incredibly rewarding.

• Crafting can be meditative and relaxing, providing a break from the fast-paced digital world. It allows you to focus on the present moment and enjoy the tactile experience of working with materials.

• Handmade items often have a special meaning for both the creator and the recipient. They can be personalized gifts that express care and thoughtfulness.

Engage in crafting activities as a form of self-expression and relaxation.

• Choose crafting projects that resonate with your personal style and interests. This can be a great way to explore your creativity and develop new skills.

• Set aside dedicated time for crafting to unwind and de-stress. The repetitive motions of activities like knitting or crocheting can be soothing and help clear your mind.

• Don't worry about perfection. The beauty of handmade items lies in their imperfections and the unique touch of the creator.

Share your creations and connect with a crafting community.

• Sharing your craft projects with others can be a source of pride and joy. It can also inspire others to try their hand at crafting.

• Join online forums, social media groups, or local clubs to connect with fellow crafters. These communities can offer support, inspiration, and a sense of belonging.

• Participating in craft fairs or selling your creations online can be a way to share your work with a wider audience and even turn your hobby into a small business.

By incorporating music, dance, crafting, and DIY projects into your life, you can experience the emotional uplift, joy, and satisfaction from creative expression and meaningful engagement with the arts.

Cooking and Baking

Experiencing the joy of preparing meals and treats.

• Cooking and baking can be a delightful and fulfilling way to express creativity and nourish the body and soul. Preparing food offers a sensory experience, from the aroma of fresh ingredients to the stove's warmth.

• Whether you're a seasoned chef or a beginner in the kitchen, cooking or baking can bring a sense of accomplishment and joy. It's a chance to experiment with flavors, textures, and presentation.

• Cooking and baking can also be a form of self-care, providing an opportunity to unwind and focus on the task. There's a special satisfaction in turning raw ingredients into a delicious meal or treat.

Experiment with new recipes and share them with loved ones.

• One of the pleasures of cooking and baking is the endless variety of recipes to explore. Challenge yourself to try new dishes, ingredients, or cooking techniques to keep things exciting and expand your culinary skills.

• Share your culinary creations with family and friends. Cooking for others can be a way to show love and care, and sharing meals is a time-honored way to connect and create memories.

• Document your favorite recipes and the stories behind them. This can be a way to pass down family traditions or create a personal collection of tried-and-true dishes.

Host cooking or baking sessions to foster creativity and connection.

• Organize cooking or baking sessions with friends or family members. This can be a fun way to spend time together, learn from each other, and enjoy the fruits of your labor.

• Consider themed cooking nights, such as a pizza-making party or a bake-off challenge, to add an element of excitement and friendly competition.

• Use these sessions as an opportunity to share tips, techniques, and cultural traditions. Cooking and baking together can be a way to explore different cuisines and celebrate diversity through food.

By embracing the joys of cooking and baking, you can experience the satisfaction of creating delicious meals and treats, connect with loved ones, and cultivate a sense of creativity and well-being in the kitchen.

CHAPTER 3

Fostering Connections and Community

"Happiness is only real when shared." - Christopher McCandless.

Building Meaningful Relationships

Prioritize quality time with family and friends.

• In the hustle and bustle of daily life, it's important to carve out time specifically for connecting with family and friends. Quality time is not just about being in the same space but about being present and engaged with each other.

• Plan regular activities or outings that allow you to spend meaningful time together. This could be as simple as a weekly family dinner, a monthly game night with friends, or an annual vacation.

• Use this time to create shared experiences and memories. Whether trying a new hobby together, exploring a new place, or just having a heartfelt conversation, these moments can strengthen your bonds and enrich your relationships.

Engage in activities that strengthen bonds.

• Participate in activities that require teamwork and cooperation, such as sports, group projects, or volunteering. These experiences can foster a sense of unity and collaboration.

• Celebrate each other's successes and support each other through challenges. Being there for one another in both good and bad can deepen your connections and build trust.

• Create traditions or rituals that are unique to your relationship. These could be annual events, special celebrations, or even small daily or weekly habits that you look forward to.

Practice active listening and empathy to deepen connections.

• Active listening involves giving the speaker your full attention, acknowledging their feelings, and responding thoughtfully. This shows that you value their perspective and are genuinely interested in what they have to say.

• Empathy is the ability to understand and share the feelings of another. Put yourself in their shoes and offer compassion and support. This can create a safe space for open and honest communication.

• Regularly check in with your loved ones to see how they're doing. Ask about their experiences, thoughts, and feelings, and share your own. This mutual exchange can foster a deeper emotional connection and a stronger sense of belonging.

You can build meaningful and lasting relationships with family and friends by prioritizing quality time, engaging in bond-strengthening activities, and practicing active listening and empathy. These connections are the foundation of a supportive and loving community.

Volunteering and Giving Back

Discover the happiness that comes from helping others.

• Volunteering and giving back to the community are powerful ways to find purpose and joy in life. Helping others can provide a sense of fulfillment and satisfaction that is difficult to find elsewhere.

• Studies have shown that engaging in acts of kindness and generosity can increase happiness, reduce stress, and give a greater sense of well-being. The positive emotions associated with altruism, known as the "helper's high," can impact one's mood and outlook on life.

• By contributing to the well-being of others, you can also foster a sense of connectedness and belonging. Helping others can remind you of the shared humanity and interdependence among all people.

Get involved in community service or volunteer work.

• Identify causes or organizations that align with your values and interests. These could include environmental conservation, supporting older people, or working with children.

• Look for volunteer opportunities in your local community, such as at food banks, shelters, schools, or community centers. Even a few hours of your time can make a significant difference.

• Consider using your skills and talents to contribute meaningfully. For example, if you're good at cooking, you could volunteer to prepare meals for a soup kitchen. If you're an artist, you could offer to teach a free class at a community center.

Reflect on the impact of your contributions and the joy it brings.

• Take time to reflect on your volunteering efforts' positive impact on others and yourself. Recognize the difference you're making in the lives of those you help.

• Celebrate the successes and learn from the challenges you encounter in your volunteer work. This can help you grow and find even more fulfillment in your efforts.

• Share your experiences with friends and family to inspire them to get involved and spread the joy of giving back. Doing so can create a ripple effect of kindness and positivity in your community.

Volunteering and giving back not only benefit those you help but also enrich your own life. The happiness that comes from helping others is a profound and rewarding experience that can lead to deeper connections, personal growth, and a more meaningful life.

Joining Clubs or Groups

It is finding communities that share your interests or hobbies.

• Joining clubs or groups that align with your interests or hobbies is a great way to connect with like-minded individuals. Whether it's a book club, a gardening group, a sports team, or an art collective, being part of a community can enhance your sense of belonging and identity.

• Look for local clubs or online communities that cater to your interests. Libraries, community centers, and social media platforms can be good places to start your search.

• Don't hesitate to step out of your comfort zone and try something new. Joining a group slightly outside your usual interests can broaden your horizons and introduce you to new experiences and perspectives.

Participate in group activities and events.

• Actively participating in group activities and events can deepen your connection with the community and enrich your experience. Attend meetings, workshops, social gatherings, and other events the group organizes.

• Volunteer to help with group projects or events. This can be a way to contribute to the group's success and show your commitment and enthusiasm.

• Engage in discussions, share your ideas and experiences, and collaborate with others. The exchange of knowledge and skills can be mutually beneficial and foster a supportive and dynamic environment.

Form new friendships and support networks.

• Joining clubs or groups can provide opportunities to form new friendships and build support networks. These connections can offer emotional support, advice, and camaraderie.

• Be open to connecting with people from diverse backgrounds and walks of life. This can enrich your social circle and provide a broader perspective on the world.

• Nurture these friendships by staying in touch, offering support, and making an effort to spend time together outside of group activities. Strong friendships can provide stability and belonging that enhance your overall well-being.

By joining clubs or groups that align with your interests, actively participating in activities, and forming new friendships, you can enrich your social life and create a supportive community that enhances your happiness and fulfillment.

Hosting Gatherings

Planning and hosting small get-togethers or parties.

• Hosting gatherings is a wonderful way to strengthen bonds with family and friends and create community. Start by choosing a theme or occasion for your get-together, such as a dinner party, game night, or seasonal celebration.

• Plan the details of your event, including the guest list, menu, decorations, and activities. Consider the preferences and needs of your guests to ensure everyone feels welcome and comfortable.

• Send out invitations well in advance, and keep your guests informed about any important details or changes. Good communication is key to a successful gathering.

Create memorable experiences for your guests.

• Focus on creating an atmosphere that encourages relaxation, conversation, and enjoyment. This could involve setting up cozy seating areas, playing background music, or incorporating fun icebreakers.

• Personal touches can make your gathering more memorable. Consider adding thoughtful details like personalized place cards, a signature cocktail, or a homemade dessert.

• Be attentive to your guests' needs during the event. Make sure everyone feels included and has a good time. Your warmth and hospitality will leave a lasting impression.

Enjoy the process of bringing people together.

• While hosting can involve some work, try to enjoy the process of bringing people together. The joy of connecting with loved ones and creating shared experiences is what makes it all worthwhile.

• Don't strive for perfection. Remember that the goal is to have fun and enjoy each other's company. Embrace any imperfections or unexpected moments as part of the experience.

• Take a moment during the gathering to appreciate the connections being made and the memories being created. The sense of community and belonging that comes from hosting can be deeply rewarding.

By planning and hosting small gatherings, you can create memorable experiences for your guests and enjoy the process of bringing people together. These events can strengthen bonds, foster a sense of community, and enrich your social life.

Connecting with Nature

Spend time outdoors to feel more connected to the world.

• Spending time in nature has numerous benefits for physical and mental well-being. It can reduce stress, improve mood, and enhance feelings of connectedness to the world.

• Make a conscious effort to spend time outdoors regularly. Even a short walk in a park or sitting in a garden can help you feel more grounded and present.

• Allow yourself to experience the natural surroundings fully. Pay attention to the sights, sounds, and smells. Feel the sun on your skin, the breeze in your hair, and the earth beneath your feet.

Engage in activities like gardening, hiking, or birdwatching.

• Engaging in outdoor activities can deepen your connection with nature and provide a sense of accomplishment and joy. Gardening allows you to work with the earth and witness the growth of plants and flowers.

• Hiking in natural settings can be a great way to explore the beauty of the landscape and challenge yourself physically. It's an opportunity to appreciate the diversity of ecosystems and the tranquility of the wilderness.

• Birdwatching is a peaceful and rewarding activity that can help you develop a greater appreciation for wildlife and the intricate balance of nature.

Observing and learning about different bird species encourages mindfulness and patience.

Appreciate the beauty and serenity of nature.

• Take the time to appreciate the simple yet profound beauty of the natural world. Notice the intricate patterns of leaves, the vibrant colors of flowers, and the majestic landscapes of mountains and forests.

• Embrace the serenity and peace that nature offers. The serenity of natural settings can provide a respite from the noise and busyness of everyday life, allowing you to recharge and find inner calm.

• Cultivate gratitude for the natural world and its wonders. Recognize the interdependence of all living things and the importance of preserving the environment for future generations.

Connecting with nature is a powerful way to enhance your well-being, foster a sense of wonder, and deepen your appreciation for the world. You can cultivate a more mindful and harmonious relationship with the natural world by spending time outdoors and engaging in nature-based activities.

CHAPTER 4

Embracing Simplicity and Decluttering

"Simplicity is the ultimate sophistication." - Leonardo da Vinci.

The Joy of Minimalism

Understand the principles of minimalism and its benefits.

• Minimalism is a lifestyle choice that emphasizes living with less to create more space for what truly matters. It's about prioritizing quality over quantity and finding contentment in simplicity.

• The benefits of minimalism include reduced stress, increased clarity and focus, and a greater sense of freedom. By eliminating excess, you can create more room for experiences, relationships, and activities that bring you joy and fulfillment.

• Minimalism encourages mindfulness and intentional living. It's about making conscious choices about what you own and how you spend your time, leading to a more purposeful and satisfying life.

Learn to let go of unnecessary possessions.

• Decluttering is a key aspect of minimalism. Start by evaluating your belongings and identifying what is truly necessary and meaningful to you.

• Let go of items that no longer serve a purpose or bring you joy. This can include clothes you don't wear, gadgets you don't use, or sentimental items stored away and forgotten.

• Remember that releasing physical possessions can also lead to emotional release. It's an opportunity to let go of past attachments and make space for new experiences and growth.

Create a peaceful and clutter-free living space.

• A minimalist living space is characterized by simplicity, cleanliness, and order. Aim to create a calm and inviting environment, with only the essentials on display.

• Organize your belongings so they are easy to access and maintain. Use storage solutions that are both functional and aesthetically pleasing.

• Regularly reassess your living space and make adjustments as needed. Minimalism is an ongoing process of refining and simplifying your environment to reflect your current needs and values.

Embracing minimalism can lead to a more peaceful and clutter-free living space and a deeper sense of contentment and well-being. By understanding the principles of minimalism, learning to let go of unnecessary possessions, and creating a simplified living environment, you can experience the joy and freedom that come with living a minimalist lifestyle.

Mindful Consumption

Reflect on your purchasing habits and their impact on happiness.

• Take time to examine your buying habits and consider whether they align with your values and contribute to your happiness. Ask yourself if your purchases are driven by need, desire, or external pressures.

• Consider the long-term impact of your purchases on your well-being and life satisfaction. Are they adding value to your life or contributing to clutter and stress?

• Reflect on the emotional triggers that may lead to impulse buying, such as seeking comfort or trying to keep up with social trends. Acknowledge these feelings and explore healthier ways to address them.

Practice conscious consumerism by buying only what you need.

• Adopt a more intentional approach to shopping by focusing on purchasing necessary and truly meaningful items. This can help reduce waste, save money, and simplify your life.

• Before making a purchase, pause and consider if the item is something you truly need and will use regularly. Ask yourself if it aligns with your values and if more sustainable or ethical alternatives are available.

• Embrace the concept of "less is more" by investing in quality items that are built to last rather than accumulating a large quantity of cheaper, disposable goods. This can lead to a more sustainable and fulfilling lifestyle.

Appreciate the value of experiences over material possessions.

• Shift your focus from acquiring material possessions to creating and enjoying meaningful experiences. Research has shown that experiences, rather than things, are more likely to lead to lasting happiness.

• Invest in activities that enrich your life, such as traveling, learning new skills, or spending quality time with loved ones. These experiences can create memories and connections that are far more valuable than physical objects.

• Cultivate gratitude for your experiences and opportunities, rather than constantly seeking new possessions. This can lead to a greater sense of contentment and appreciation for what you already have.

Adopting mindful consumption can lead to a more intentional and satisfying lifestyle. Reflecting on your purchasing habits, focusing on buying only what you need, and valuing experiences over material possessions can lead to a deeper sense of happiness and fulfillment.

Decluttering Your Space

Implement decluttering strategies for a more organized home.

• Begin your decluttering journey by tackling one area or room at a time. This will prevent you from feeling overwhelmed and allow you to see progress quickly.

• Sort through your belongings using the "keep, donate, discard" method. Be honest with yourself about what items you truly need, use, and love.

• Consider implementing the "one in, one out" rule to maintain a clutter-free space. Whenever you bring a new item into your home, let go of something else to prevent accumulation.

Experience the mental clarity that comes from a tidy environment.

• A decluttered and organized space can lead to a clearer mind and reduced stress. When your environment is clutter-free, it's easier to focus, make decisions, and feel at peace.

• Notice how a tidy space can improve your mood and productivity. A well-organized environment can inspire creativity and motivation, making tackling daily tasks and goals easier.

• Embrace the simplicity of a decluttered home. A minimalist space can promote a sense of calm and contentment, allowing you to enjoy the beauty of simplicity.

Donate or repurpose items to extend their usefulness and joy.

• When decluttering, consider donating items that are still in good condition to charity or giving them to friends or family who can use them. This not only clears your space but also helps others in need.

• Repurpose items instead of discarding them. For example, an old jar can become a vase or a worn-out t-shirt can be transformed into a cleaning rag. This approach is both environmentally friendly and creative.

• Reflect on the joy that your items can bring to others. By passing them on, you're decluttering your own space and spreading happiness and usefulness to someone else's life.

Decluttering your space is a transformative process that can lead to a more organized home, mental clarity, and a deeper appreciation for the items you choose to keep. By implementing decluttering strategies, experiencing the benefits of a tidy environment, and thoughtfully donating or repurposing items, you can create a living space that reflects simplicity, mindfulness, and joy.

Simplifying Your Schedule

Assess and prioritize your commitments for a balanced life.

• Take a close look at your current schedule and commitments. Make a list of all your regular activities, responsibilities, and obligations.

• Evaluate each item on your list based on its importance, value, and alignment with your personal goals and values. Prioritize tasks and commitments that are essential and meaningful to you.

• Consider which commitments can be delegated, rescheduled, or eliminated altogether. Simplifying your schedule involves making tough choices about what truly deserves your time and energy.

Learn to say no to activities that don't bring you joy.

• One key aspect of simplifying your schedule is learning to say no to invitations, requests, and activities that don't align with your priorities or bring you joy.

• Practice setting boundaries and communicating your decisions respectfully but firmly. Deciding opportunities that don't fit into your simplified lifestyle is okay.

• Remember that saying no to one thing allows you to say yes to something else that may be more fulfilling or important to you.

Make time for relaxation and self-care.

• In your pursuit of a balanced life, ensure that

you allocate time for relaxation and self-care. These are essential components of a healthy and simplified schedule.

• Schedule regular breaks, downtime, and leisure activities just as you would any other commitment. Treat these moments as non-negotiable appointments with yourself.

• Engage in activities that rejuvenate your mind, body, and spirit. Whether reading a book, taking a bath, practicing meditation, or spending time in nature, find what helps you unwind and prioritize it in your schedule.

By assessing and prioritizing your commitments, learning to say no to activities that don't bring you joy, and making time for relaxation and self-care, you can simplify your schedule and create a more balanced and fulfilling life. This approach allows you to focus on what truly matters and ensures that your time is spent in a way that aligns with your values and goals.

Digital Detox

Recognize the importance of unplugging from technology.

• In today's digital age, it's easy to become overwhelmed by the constant barrage of notifications, emails, and social media updates. Recognizing the importance of unplugging from technology is the first step toward creating a more balanced and mindful life.

• Excessive screen time can lead to digital burnout, decreased productivity, and a sense of disconnection from the physical world. Taking regular breaks from digital devices can help you recharge and refocus.

• Consider the impact of technology on your mental and emotional well-being. Unplugging can reduce stress, improve sleep, and enhance your overall sense of happiness and contentment.

Set boundaries for screen time and social media use.

• Establish clear boundaries for when and how you use your digital devices. This might include designated tech-free times, such as during meals, before bed, or on weekends.

• Use tools and apps that help you monitor and limit your screen time. Many smartphones now offer features that track your usage and allow you to set daily limits for specific apps.

• Be intentional about your social media consumption. Curate your feeds to include content that is positive, inspiring, and aligned with your values. Unfollow or mute accounts that contribute to feelings of negativity or comparison.

Reconnect with real-life experiences and interactions.

• Use the time you gain from unplugging to engage in activities that enrich your life and bring you joy. This could include spending time with loved ones, pursuing hobbies, or exploring the outdoors.

• Cultivate face-to-face interactions and build meaningful relationships. In-person connections can provide a deeper sense of community and support than digital ones.

• Embrace the beauty of the present moment. Without the distraction of devices, you can fully immerse yourself in your surroundings and experiences, leading to a more fulfilling and mindful life.

By recognizing the importance of a digital detox, setting boundaries for technology use, and reconnecting with real-life experiences, you can simplify your digital life and create space for more meaningful and rewarding activities. This balance can lead to greater well-being and a deeper appreciation for the world around you.

CHAPTER 5

Cultivating Personal Growth and Learning

"The capacity to learn is a gift; the ability to learn is a skill; the willingness to learn is a choice." - Brian Herbert.

Setting and Achieving Goals

Identify personal goals that align with your values and happiness.

• Start by reflecting on your values, interests, and aspirations. Consider what truly matters to you and what you want to achieve in different areas of your life, such as career, relationships, health, and personal development.

• Set goals that are aligned with your values and contribute to your overall happiness. For example, if you value creativity, you might set a goal to complete a creative project. If health is important to you, your goal could be establishing a regular exercise routine.

• Ensure your goals are specific, measurable, achievable, relevant, and time-bound (SMART). This clarity will help you stay focused and motivated.

Break down goals into actionable steps and track your progress.

• Once you have identified your goals, break them down into smaller, manageable steps. This will make the process less overwhelming and more achievable.

• Create an action plan for each step, including deadlines and needed resources. This will help you stay organized and on track.

• Regularly monitor your progress towards your goals. Use a journal, app, or spreadsheet to track your achievements and reflect on your journey. This can provide motivation and insight into what's working and needs adjustment.

Celebrate achievements and learn from setbacks.

• Acknowledge and celebrate your accomplishments, no matter how small. This will boost your confidence and motivation to continue pursuing your goals.

• Treat setbacks as learning opportunities. Reflect on what led to the setback, what you can learn from it, and how you can adjust your approach moving forward. Resilience is key to achieving long-term goals.

• Share your successes and challenges with supportive friends or mentors. They can offer encouragement, advice, and accountability, helping you stay committed to your goals.

By setting and achieving goals that align with your values, breaking them down into actionable steps, and celebrating achievements while learning from setbacks, you can foster personal growth and move closer to a life of happiness and fulfillment.

Lifelong Learning

Embrace curiosity and the pursuit of knowledge.

• Lifelong learning is about maintaining a curious and open mindset throughout life and continuously seeking new knowledge, skills, and experiences.

• Cultivate curiosity by asking questions, exploring new ideas, and challenging your assumptions. This will keep your mind active and engaged.

• Recognize that learning is not confined to formal education. It can occur in everyday experiences, interactions with others, and self-reflection.

Explore new subjects or skills through courses, books, or workshops.

• Take advantage of the vast resources available for learning. Enroll in online courses, attend workshops, or read books on topics that interest you.

• Don't limit yourself to subjects directly related to your career or current knowledge. Exploring diverse topics can broaden your perspective and lead to unexpected insights and opportunities.

• Practice hands-on learning whenever possible. Whether it's a new hobby, a language, or a professional skill, applying what you learn in practical ways can enhance understanding and retention.

Share your learning experiences with others to inspire and motivate.

• Sharing your learning journey with others can be mutually beneficial. It can reinforce your own knowledge and provide valuable insights to others.

• Consider writing a blog, participating in discussion groups, or giving presentations on what you've learned. Teaching is one of the most effective ways to deepen your understanding of a subject.

• Encourage a culture of learning in your community or workplace. Share resources, exchange ideas, and collaborate on learning projects. This can create a supportive environment that fosters growth and innovation.

Embracing lifelong learning is a key component of personal growth. By staying curious, exploring new subjects and skills, and sharing your learning experiences, you can continue to evolve and enrich your life.

Self-Reflection and Journaling

Practice regular self-reflection to gain insights into your happiness.

• Self-reflection is the process of examining one's thoughts, feelings, and behaviors to gain a deeper understanding of oneself and one's life. It can be a powerful tool for personal growth and happiness.

• Set aside time each day or week for quiet reflection. Consider what brings you joy, what challenges you face, and what you are grateful for. This can help you stay aligned with your values and goals.

• Use reflection to identify areas for improvement and celebrate your successes. Acknowledging your achievements, no matter how small can boost your confidence and motivation.

Use journaling as a tool for personal growth and emotional release.

• Journaling is a practical and effective way to engage in self-reflection. Writing down your thoughts and feelings can help you process emotions, clarify your thoughts, and gain perspective.

• Experiment with different journaling techniques, such as gratitude journaling, stream-of-consciousness writing, or keeping a daily diary. Find what works best for you and your personal growth journey.

• Review your journal entries periodically to track your progress and identify patterns in your thoughts and behaviors. This can provide valuable insights and guide your future actions.

Set intentions and affirmations to guide your journey.

• Setting intentions is a powerful way to focus your mind and direct your energy toward your desired outcomes. Each morning, take a moment to set a clear intention for the day, such as being kind to yourself or staying focused on your goals.

• Use affirmations to reinforce positive beliefs and attitudes. Repeat positive statements to yourself, such as "I am capable of achieving my goals" or "I am worthy of happiness." Affirmations can help you cultivate a positive mindset and overcome self-doubt.

• Regularly revisit and adjust your intentions and affirmations as you grow and evolve. They can serve as guiding lights on your path to personal growth and happiness.

By practicing self-reflection, journaling as a tool for personal growth, and setting intentions and affirmations, you can gain deeper insights into your happiness and continue evolving on your journey toward a fulfilling life.

Overcoming Challenges

Develop resilience and coping strategies for life's obstacles.

• Resilience is the ability to bounce back from setbacks and challenges. Developing resilience involves cultivating a positive mindset, practicing flexibility, and managing stress effectively.

• Identify coping strategies that work for you, such as engaging in physical activity, seeking solace in nature, practicing mindfulness, or using creative outlets like writing or art. These strategies can help you navigate difficult times with greater ease.

• Remember that resilience is built over time through experiences. Each challenge you face and overcome contributes to your ability to handle future obstacles more effectively.

Learn from challenges and view them as opportunities for growth.

• Adopting a growth mindset means seeing challenges not as insurmountable barriers but as opportunities to learn, develop, and grow. This perspective can transform the way you approach difficulties.

• After facing a challenge, reflect on what you've learned from the experience. Ask yourself what skills you developed, how you adapted, and what you might do differently in the future.

• Recognize that growth often comes from discomfort. Stepping out of your comfort zone and facing challenges head-on can lead to significant personal development and a deeper understanding of yourself.

Seek support and guidance when needed to navigate tough times.

• It's important to know that you don't have to face challenges alone. Seeking support from friends, family, mentors, or professionals can provide comfort, advice, and different perspectives.

• Join support groups or communities where you can share experiences and learn from others who have faced similar challenges. There's strength in shared experiences and collective wisdom.

• Consider professional guidance, such as counseling or coaching, if you're struggling to overcome a particular challenge. Professionals can offer strategies, tools, and support tailored to your specific needs.

Overcoming challenges is an integral part of personal growth and development. By developing resilience, learning from your experiences, and seeking support when needed, you can navigate life's obstacles more effectively and emerge stronger and wiser.

Embracing Change

Cultivate a positive attitude towards change and uncertainty.

• Change and uncertainty are inevitable parts of life. Cultivating a positive attitude towards them can help you navigate these challenges gracefully and be resilient.

• Practice mindfulness and acceptance to stay grounded in the present moment, even when faced with uncertainty. This can help you remain calm and open to the possibilities that change can bring.

• Reframe your perspective on change by viewing it as an opportunity for growth and learning. Embrace the idea that change can lead to new experiences, insights, and personal development.

Adapt to new situations and find joy in the unknown.

• Being adaptable is a valuable skill in times of change. Cultivate flexibility in your thoughts and actions to adjust to new circumstances more easily.

• Approach new situations with curiosity and a sense of adventure. Finding joy in the unknown can make transitions more exciting and less daunting.

• Stay connected to your core values and goals, even adapting to change. This can provide a sense of continuity and purpose amidst uncertainty.

Recognize that growth often comes from embracing change.

• Personal growth often results from stepping

out of your comfort zone and embracing change. Reflect on past experiences where change has led to positive outcomes and personal development.

• Set intentions for growth and learning as you navigate life changes. Use challenges as opportunities to strengthen your character, acquire new skills, and gain a deeper understanding of yourself and the world around you.

• Celebrate your progress and growth as you embrace change. Acknowledge the courage and resilience it takes to adapt to new situations and use these experiences to build confidence in your ability to handle future changes.

By cultivating a positive attitude towards change, adapting to new situations with joy, and recognizing the growth that comes from embracing change, you can navigate life's uncertainties with confidence and resilience. This mindset can lead to a more fulfilling and dynamic life, enriched by the opportunities and lessons that change brings.

CHAPTER 6

Finding Balance and Harmony in Life

"Life is all about balance. You don't always need to be getting stuff done. Sometimes it's perfectly okay, and absolutely necessary, to shut down, kick back, and do nothing." - Lori Deschene.

Work-Life Balance

Assess your current work-life balance and identify areas for improvement.

• Begin by evaluating how you currently allocate your time and energy between work and personal life. Are there areas where you feel overwhelmed or neglected?

• Reflect on how your work-life balance affects your well-being, relationships, and overall satisfaction with life. Consider any signs of burnout, stress, or disconnection from personal interests and relationships.

• Identify specific areas for improvement, such as reducing work hours, delegating tasks, or making more time for leisure and family activities.

Set boundaries between work and personal time.

• Establish clear boundaries to separate your work life from your personal life. This might include setting specific work hours, turning off work-related notifications after hours, and having a dedicated workspace if you work from home.

• Communicate your boundaries to colleagues, clients, and family members to ensure they are respected. Be firm but polite in enforcing these limits to protect your personal time.

• Practice discipline in adhering to your boundaries. Avoid checking work emails or taking work calls during your designated personal time, and vice versa.

Prioritize activities that contribute to your overall well-being.

• Make a conscious effort to prioritize activities that enhance your physical, emotional, and mental well-being. This could include regular exercise, hobbies, socializing with loved ones, and relaxation practices.

• Schedule these activities into your day or week as non-negotiable appointments, just like you would with work commitments. Please treat them with the same importance to ensure they are not overlooked.

• Regularly reassess your priorities to ensure your work-life balance aligns with your values and goals. Be willing to make adjustments as needed to maintain a healthy and fulfilling balance.

Achieving a healthy work-life balance is crucial for maintaining well-being, preventing burnout, and ensuring satisfaction in both personal and professional aspects of life. You can create a more harmonious and fulfilling life by assessing your current balance, setting clear boundaries, and prioritizing activities contributing to your overall well-being.

Stress Management

Understand the impact of stress on happiness and health.

• Recognize that stress is a natural response to challenging situations, but chronic stress can have negative effects on both mental and physical health. It can lead to anxiety, depression, cardiovascular diseases, and weakened immune systems, among other issues.

• Acknowledge the importance of managing stress to maintain overall happiness and well-being. Unmanaged stress can strain relationships, reduce productivity, and diminish the quality of life.

• Identify the sources of stress in your life, whether they are work-related, personal, or a combination of both. Understanding the root causes is the first step in developing effective stress management strategies.

Learn relaxation techniques such as deep breathing, meditation, or yoga.

• Deep breathing exercises can help calm the mind and reduce tension in the body. Practice taking slow, deep breaths, focusing on filling your lungs and exhaling fully.

• Meditation is a powerful tool for cultivating mindfulness and reducing stress. Start with short, guided meditations and gradually increase the duration as you become more comfortable with the practice.

• Yoga combines physical postures, breathing exercises, and meditation to promote relaxation and stress relief. Consider joining a yoga class or following online tutorials to incorporate yoga into your routine.

Develop a personal stress management plan.

• Create a personalized plan that includes a variety of stress-reducing activities and techniques. These might include regular exercise, spending time in nature, engaging in hobbies, or practicing relaxation methods like those mentioned above.

• Set aside dedicated time each day for stress-reducing activities. Make this a non-negotiable part of your routine, like eating or sleeping.

• Be proactive in addressing stress. If you anticipate a stressful situation, prepare by using your stress management techniques beforehand. After a stressful event, take time to unwind and reset.

Effective stress management is essential for maintaining happiness and health. By understanding the impact of stress, learning relaxation techniques, and developing a personal stress management plan, you can better navigate life's challenges and enjoy a more balanced and fulfilling life.

Physical Wellness

Recognize the connection between physical health and happiness.

• Understand that physical health and mental well-being are closely linked. A healthy body can support a healthy mind, increasing happiness, energy, and resilience.

• Regular physical activity and a balanced diet can improve mood, reduce stress and anxiety, and boost self-esteem. Conversely, poor physical health can contribute to feelings of depression and lower life satisfaction.

• Pay attention to how your body feels and responds to different lifestyle choices. This awareness can guide you in making decisions that support your physical and emotional well-being.

Incorporate regular exercise and healthy eating into your lifestyle.

• Make physical activity a regular part of your routine. Aim for at least 150 minutes of moderate aerobic exercise or 75 minutes of vigorous exercise each week, along with muscle-strengthening activities on two or more days.

• Choose a form of exercise you enjoy, whether walking, cycling, swimming, dancing, or any other activity that gets you moving. This will make it easier to stick to your routine.

• Focus on a balanced diet that includes a variety of fruits, vegetables, whole grains, lean proteins, and healthy fats. Pay attention to portion sizes and try to limit processed foods and added sugars.

Get adequate rest and prioritize sleep for overall well-being.

• Recognize the importance of sleep in maintaining physical health and emotional balance. Aim for 7-9 hours of quality sleep each night.

• Establish a regular sleep schedule by going to bed and waking up at the same time every day, even on weekends. This can help regulate your body's internal clock and improve the quality of your sleep.

• Create a relaxing bedtime routine to signal your body that it's time to wind down. This might include reading, taking a warm bath, or practicing relaxation techniques.

Recognizing the connection between physical health and happiness, incorporating regular exercise and healthy eating into your lifestyle, and prioritizing sleep can enhance your physical wellness and contribute to a more balanced and fulfilling life.

Emotional Wellness

Cultivate emotional intelligence and self-awareness.

• Emotional intelligence involves recognizing, understanding, and managing your own emotions, as well as empathizing with the emotions of others. It's a key component of emotional wellness.

• Develop self-awareness by regularly reflecting on your emotions and reactions. Ask yourself why you feel a certain way and how your emotions influence your thoughts and behaviors.

• Enhance your emotional intelligence by practicing active listening, empathy, and effective communication in your interactions with others. This can lead to healthier relationships and a deeper understanding of yourself and those around you.

Practice self-compassion and kindness towards yourself and others.

• Treat yourself with the kindness and understanding you would offer a friend. Acknowledge that everyone has flaws and makes mistakes, and avoid harsh self-criticism.

• Engage in positive self-talk and affirmations to boost your self-esteem and confidence. Remind yourself of your strengths and accomplishments.

• Extend compassion and kindness to others. This can foster a sense of connection and community, which are important for emotional well-being.

Acts of kindness can also boost your mood and create a positive feedback loop of goodwill.

Seek professional help if needed for emotional or mental health issues.

• Recognize that seeking help for emotional or mental health issues is a sign of strength, not weakness. If you're struggling to cope with your emotions or facing mental health challenges, reaching out for support can be a crucial step towards healing.

• Consult a mental health professional, such as a therapist or counselor, for guidance and support. They can provide strategies and tools to help you manage your emotions and work through challenges.

• Don't hesitate to seek help if you're experiencing symptoms of depression, anxiety, or other mental health conditions. Early intervention can lead to better outcomes and improve your overall quality of life.

Emotional wellness is a vital aspect of overall well-being. By cultivating emotional intelligence and self-awareness, practicing self-compassion and kindness, and seeking professional help when needed, you can build a strong foundation for a balanced and fulfilling life.

Spiritual Wellness

Explore your spiritual beliefs and practices.

• Spiritual wellness involves exploring and understanding your own beliefs, values, and ethics. It's about finding meaning and purpose in life, which may or may not relate to a specific religion or spiritual practice.

• Take time to reflect on what spirituality means to you. This could involve nature, art, meditation, religion, or personal growth. Exploring various spiritual practices can help you discover what resonates with you and provides a sense of peace and grounding.

• Keep an open mind and heart as you explore different spiritual paths. Reading, attending workshops, or speaking with others about their spiritual experiences can provide insights and inspiration.

Find solace and happiness in spirituality or mindfulness.

• Many people find that engaging in spiritual or mindfulness practices brings them comfort, happiness, and a deeper connection to themselves and the world around them.

• Practices such as meditation, prayer, yoga, or mindfulness exercises can help reduce stress, improve mental clarity, and foster a sense of inner peace.

• Spirituality and mindfulness can also enhance your awareness of the present moment, encouraging gratitude and a deeper appreciation for life's experiences.

Connect with a community or group that shares your spiritual values.

• Joining a community or group that shares your spiritual beliefs or interests can provide a sense of belonging, support, and shared purpose. This could be a religious congregation, meditation group, yoga class, or spiritual study group.

• Participating in community rituals, ceremonies, or discussions can enrich your spiritual journey and provide personal reflection and growth opportunities.

• Be respectful and open to learning from others, even if their beliefs differ from yours. The diversity of spiritual experiences can broaden your understanding and appreciation of the many ways people find meaning and connection in their lives.

Spiritual wellness is a deeply personal aspect of overall well-being, encompassing a wide range of beliefs and practices. By exploring your spiritual beliefs, finding solace in spirituality or mindfulness, and connecting with a like-minded community, you can nurture your spiritual wellness and enhance your life's richness and depth.

CHAPTER 7

Savoring Life's Simple Pleasures

"Sometimes the simplest things are the most profound." - Carolina Herrera.

Appreciating the Small Moments

Learn to recognize and savor the joy in everyday moments.

• Cultivate an attitude of mindfulness and gratitude to notice the beauty and joy in ordinary moments. This could be the sound of birds singing, the smell of freshly baked bread, or the feeling of a gentle breeze.

• Slow down and take the time to experience these moments fully. Please pay attention to the details and sensations and appreciate the simple pleasures they offer.

• Reflect on the positive aspects of your day, no matter how small. This practice can shift your focus from what's lacking to what's abundant in your life.

Practice being present and fully engaged in the here and now.

• Being present means giving your full attention to the current moment without being distracted by thoughts of the past or worries about the future. It allows you to experience life more fully and deeply.

• Engage all your senses to immerse yourself in the present. For example, notice your food's flavors, textures, and colors when eating. When listening to music, focus on the different instruments and rhythms.

• Use mindfulness techniques, such as deep breathing or body scans, to center yourself in the present moment, especially when you feel your mind wandering.

Cherish simple pleasures like a warm cup of tea or a beautiful sunset.

• Simple pleasures are often the most meaningful and accessible sources of joy. They remind us that happiness can be found in the everyday and ordinary.

• Create small rituals around these pleasures to enhance your appreciation.

Laughter and Humor

Embrace the healing power of laughter and humor.

• Recognize that laughter is a source of joy and a powerful tool for improving mental and physical health. It can reduce stress, boost the immune system, and even relieve pain.

• Seek opportunities to laugh, whether engaging with humorous content, recalling funny memories, or simply not taking yourself too seriously.

• Remember that humor is subjective. What makes you laugh may not be the same for someone else. Embrace your unique sense of humor and the joy it brings to your life.

Incorporate fun and playfulness into your daily routine.

• Integrate playfulness into your daily activities to add a sense of lightness and joy to your routine. This could be as simple as dancing while you do chores or making a game out of mundane tasks.

• Surround yourself with people who make you laugh and feel good. Spending time with friends and family who have a good sense of humor can uplift your spirits and strengthen your relationships.

• Don't be afraid to be silly or playful. Engaging in childlike activities like playing with pets or drawing can reignite your sense of wonder and amusement.

Share jokes and funny stories, or watch comedies to lighten your mood.

• Sharing laughter with others can create bonding experiences and foster a sense of connection. Exchange jokes or funny stories with friends, family, or coworkers to spread joy and laughter.

• Make time to watch comedies or listen to humorous podcasts. These can provide a welcome escape from the seriousness of daily life and help you relax and unwind.

• Use humor to cope with challenges. Finding humor in difficult situations can provide a different perspective and make problems seem more manageable.

Laughter and humor are essential components of a joyful and balanced life. By embracing the healing power of laughter, incorporating fun into your routine, and sharing humorous moments with others, you can enhance your overall well-being and bring more happiness into your life.

Acts of Kindness

Experience the happiness that comes from being kind to others.

• Acts of kindness not only benefit the recipient but also the giver. Engaging in kind behavior can boost your mood, increase feelings of self-worth, and foster a sense of connection with others.

• Kindness can take many forms, from offering a helping hand to someone in need to simply offering a smile or a word of encouragement. Every act of kindness, no matter how small, contributes to a more positive and compassionate world.

• Studies have shown that kindness is contagious. Your acts of kindness can inspire others to act kindly, in turn creating a ripple effect of positivity and goodwill.

Perform random acts of kindness without expecting anything in return.

• Random acts of kindness are selfless actions performed to bring joy or assistance to others without any expectation of reward or recognition. This could be as simple as leaving a kind note for a coworker, paying for someone's coffee, or volunteering your time to help others.

• Challenge yourself to perform at least one random act of kindness daily. This can help you develop a habit of generosity and compassion.

• Remember that the value of an act of kindness lies in its intention, not in the size or grandeur of the gesture. Even the smallest acts can have a profound impact.

Notice how small gestures can make a big difference in someone's day.

• Pay attention to the impact of your kind actions. A simple gesture of kindness can brighten someone's day, provide comfort during a difficult time, or even change someone's outlook on life.

• Take note of the reactions of those you help or offer kindness to. Their smiles, gratitude, or expressions of surprise can serve as reminders of the power of kindness.

• Reflect on how acts of kindness affect your mood and well-being. Many people find that helping others brings them a sense of joy and fulfillment that is unmatched by other pursuits.

By experiencing the happiness that comes from being kind to others, performing random acts of kindness, and noticing the impact of small gestures, you can cultivate a more compassionate and fulfilling life. Acts of kindness not only enrich the lives of others but also bring immeasurable joy and satisfaction to your own.

Connection with Animals and Pets

Discover the joy and companionship that pets can bring.

• Pets can provide unconditional love, comfort, and companionship, enriching our lives in countless ways. The bond between humans and animals can be a source of immense joy and fulfillment.

• Caring for a pet can also bring structure and routine to your day, which can benefit your mental health. The responsibility of looking after an animal can instill a sense of purpose and accomplishment.

• Studies have shown that interacting with pets can reduce stress, lower blood pressure, and improve overall emotional well-being. The presence of a pet can create a sense of calm and comfort in your home.

Engage in activities like petting, walking, or playing with animals.

• Spend quality time with your pet by engaging in activities that you both enjoy. Whether going for walks, playing with toys, or simply cuddling, these moments can strengthen your bond and provide mutual enjoyment.

• Regular exercise and play are important for your pet's physical health and can be a fun way for you to stay active. For example, exploring new trails or parks with your dog can be an adventure for both of you.

• Petting and grooming your animal can be soothing activities that promote relaxation and mindfulness. The tactile experience of touching your pet can help reduce anxiety and foster a deeper connection.

Volunteer at animal shelters or consider adopting a pet.

• If you're not ready to own a pet, volunteering at an animal shelter can be a rewarding way to connect with animals and give back to your community. Shelters often need help with feeding, walking, and socializing animals.

• Volunteering can also provide valuable experience and insight into pet care, helping you make an informed decision if you're considering adoption.

• If you decide to adopt, consider choosing a rescue animal. Giving a loving home to a pet in need can be an incredibly fulfilling experience, and you'll be making a positive impact on the animal's life as well as your own.

Connecting with animals and pets offers a unique and enriching form of companionship that can bring joy, comfort, and a sense of purpose to your life. Whether through owning a pet, volunteering or simply spending time with animals, these connections can enhance your well-being and bring simple pleasures to your everyday experiences.

Enjoying Nature and the Outdoors

Reconnect with the natural world for a sense of peace and happiness.

• Spending time in nature can profoundly affect your mental and emotional well-being. The beauty and tranquility of the natural world can provide a sense of peace, awe, and happiness.

• Make a conscious effort to spend time outdoors regularly, whether it's a walk in the park, a hike in the woods, or simply sitting in your garden. These moments can help you feel more grounded and connected to the world around you.

• Allow yourself to fully immerse in the experience of being in nature. Pay attention to the sights, sounds, and smells, and let the natural beauty soothe and rejuvenate your spirit.

Take time to observe and appreciate the beauty of nature.

• Practice mindfulness while in nature by focusing on the present moment and appreciating the details around you. Notice the colors of the leaves, the patterns of the clouds, or the sound of a babbling brook.

• Take a moment to marvel at the wonders of nature, from the grandeur of a mountain range to the intricacy of a spider's web. These moments of awe can enhance your sense of gratitude and well-being.

• Capture the beauty of nature through photography, drawing, or writing. This can be a creative way to express your appreciation and create lasting memories of your experiences.

Engage in outdoor activities like gardening, picnicking, or stargazing.

• Participate in activities that allow you to interact with nature and enjoy its benefits. Gardening, for example, can be a therapeutic and rewarding way to connect with the earth and witness the cycle of life.

• Plan a picnic in a scenic location to enjoy a meal surrounded by natural beauty. This can be a delightful way to relax and spend quality time with loved ones.

• Explore the night sky through stargazing. Whether with the naked eye or a telescope, observing the stars and planets can instill a sense of wonder and remind you of the vastness and beauty of the universe.

Enjoying nature and the outdoors can provide a welcome respite from the hustle and bustle of everyday life. By reconnecting with the natural world, taking time to appreciate its beauty, and engaging in outdoor activities, you can find peace, happiness, and a deeper appreciation for the simple pleasures in life.

Embracing Creativity and Innovation

"Creativity is seeing what everyone else has seen and thinking what no one else has thought." - Albert Einstein.

Fostering a Creative Mindset

Cultivate curiosity and openness to new ideas.

• Curiosity is the fuel for creativity. Cultivate a sense of wonder and a desire to explore and understand the world around you. Ask questions, seek out new experiences, and challenge your assumptions.

• Be open to new ideas and perspectives, even if they differ from your own. This openness can lead to unexpected connections and insights that spark creative solutions.

• Surround yourself with diverse sources of inspiration, such as books, art, music, nature, or conversations with people from different backgrounds. This variety can stimulate your imagination and broaden your creative horizons.

Practice creative thinking techniques and brainstorming.

• Engage in activities encouraging creative thinking, such as brainstorming sessions, mind mapping, or free writing. These techniques can help you generate a wide range of ideas without the constraints of judgment or criticism.

• Set aside dedicated time for creativity and idea generation. This can be a regular "creative hour" where you focus solely on exploring new concepts and possibilities.

• Encourage a playful and experimental attitude during the creative process. This can help you overcome mental blocks and foster an environment where innovation can thrive.

Embrace mistakes and failures as part of the creative process.

• Recognize that mistakes and failures are inevitable and valuable learning opportunities. They provide feedback and insights that can guide your creative journey.

• Adopt a growth mindset, where you view challenges as opportunities to grow and improve rather than setbacks. This mindset can help you persist in the face of obstacles and continue to explore new avenues.

• Celebrate the risks taken and the lessons learned from failed attempts. By embracing failure as a natural part of the creative process, you can build resilience and confidence in your creative abilities.

Fostering a creative mindset is essential for innovation and personal growth. By cultivating curiosity, practicing creative thinking techniques, and embracing mistakes and failures, you can unlock your creative potential and bring fresh, innovative ideas to life.

Innovative Problem Solving

Apply creative approaches to solve everyday challenges.

• Embrace a creative mindset when faced with challenges, looking beyond conventional solutions and considering a range of possibilities. This can lead to innovative and effective ways of overcoming obstacles.

• Use techniques such as lateral thinking, which involves approaching problems from new angles, or design thinking, which focuses on empathizing with users and iterating on solutions.

• Break down larger problems into smaller, more manageable parts. This can help you identify creative solutions and prevent feeling overwhelmed.

Encourage experimentation and trying different solutions.

• Foster an environment where experimentation is encouraged, and people are willing to take calculated risks. This can lead to the discovery of new and unexpected solutions.

• Try out multiple solutions to a problem, even if some seem unconventional. This can help you find the most effective approach and spark further creativity.

• Be flexible and adaptable in your problem-solving process. If one solution doesn't work, be prepared to pivot and try another approach.

Learn from successes and failures to improve problem-solving skills.

• Reflect on the outcomes of your problem-solving efforts, analyzing what worked well and what didn't. This reflection can provide valuable insights for future challenges.

• Celebrate successes, no matter how small, as they can boost confidence and motivation. However, they also view failures as opportunities for learning and growth.

• Share your experiences and learnings with others. Collaborating and exchanging ideas can enhance your problem-solving skills and foster a culture of innovation.

Innovative problem-solving requires a combination of creative thinking, experimentation, and learning from both successes and failures. By applying these approaches to everyday challenges, you can develop more effective solutions and continuously improve your problem-solving skills.

Creative Hobbies and Projects

Explore hobbies that spark your creativity, such as painting, writing, or photography.

• Engaging in creative hobbies can provide an outlet for self-expression, relaxation, and personal fulfillment. Explore different activities to find what resonates with you and ignites your creative spark.

• Don't be afraid to try new things or combine different interests. For example, if you enjoy writing and photography, you could start a blog showcasing your photos and stories.

• Remember that the goal is not perfection but the enjoyment and satisfaction that comes from the creative process.

Set aside time for personal projects and creative pursuits.

• Prioritize creativity by scheduling regular time for your hobbies and projects. This could be a dedicated evening each week, a few hours on the weekend, or even short daily sessions.

• Create a space that inspires and supports your creativity, whether it's a corner of your room, a home studio, or a portable kit you can take.

• Use this time to experiment, explore new techniques, and fully immerse yourself in your creative endeavors without the pressure of deadlines or expectations.

Share your creations with others to inspire and be inspired.

• Sharing your work can be a rewarding experience that allows you to connect with others, receive feedback, and gain new perspectives.

• Consider showcasing your creations on social media, in local galleries or exhibitions, or through online platforms like blogs or portfolio websites.

• Engage with other creatives by attending workshops, joining clubs or online communities, or collaborating on projects. This interaction can provide motivation, inspiration, and valuable learning opportunities.

Creative hobbies and projects offer an excellent way to explore your interests, express yourself, and add a fulfilling dimension to your life. You can cultivate a rich and vibrant creative practice by setting aside time for creativity, exploring diverse activities, and sharing your work with others.

The Role of Technology in Creativity

Utilize technology and digital tools to enhance your creative expression.

• Technology offers a wide range of tools and platforms that can expand the possibilities for creative expression. Explore software, apps, and devices that cater to your specific interests, whether digital painting, music production, writing, or graphic design.

• Use technology to experiment with new techniques and styles that may not be possible with traditional methods. For example, digital art programs can allow endless editing and manipulation, providing a different creative experience than traditional painting.

• Leverage online resources and tutorials to learn how to use these tools effectively. Many platforms offer free or affordable courses to help you master digital tools and techniques.

Stay updated on technological advancements that can inspire innovation.

• Monitor emerging technologies and trends in your field of interest. Innovations such as virtual reality, augmented reality, and artificial intelligence are opening new frontiers for creative exploration.

• Attend tech conferences, follow industry blogs, or join online communities to stay informed about the latest developments and how they can be applied to your creative work.

• Consider how you can incorporate cutting-edge technology into your projects to push the boundaries of what's possible and create unique, innovative experiences.

Balance the use of technology with traditional creative methods.

• While technology can enhance creativity, it's important to maintain a balance with traditional methods. Each approach offers its own benefits and can complement the other.

• Use technology as a tool to support and enhance your creativity rather than relying on it entirely. For example, you might sketch ideas on paper before refining them digitally or use a combination of acoustic and electronic instruments in music composition.

• Take breaks from technology to engage in hands-on activities and reconnect with the tactile experience of creating. This can provide a refreshing change of pace and stimulate different aspects of your creativity.

By effectively utilizing technology and digital tools, staying updated on advancements, and balancing technology with traditional methods, you can enhance your creative expression and explore new possibilities for innovation.

Collaborating with Others

Engage in collaborative projects and activities to boost creativity.

• Collaborating with others can bring diverse perspectives, skills, and ideas to the table, leading to more innovative and creative outcomes. Look for opportunities to work on projects with people from different backgrounds or fields.

• Participate in collaborative activities such as workshops, hackathons, or group art projects. These experiences can challenge you to think differently and expand your creative horizons.

• Be open to the creative collaboration process, which may involve brainstorming, experimentation, and iteration. Embrace the dynamic nature of working with others and the potential for unexpected discoveries.

Share ideas and feedback with peers to foster a creative community.

• Create a supportive environment where ideas can be freely shared and discussed. Encourage constructive feedback and open dialogue to help each other grow and improve.

• Join or create networks, clubs, or online forums where you can connect with other creative individuals. These communities can provide inspiration, motivation, and valuable insights.

• Be generous with your knowledge and expertise. Offering guidance and support to others can strengthen the community and contribute to a culture of creativity and collaboration.

Celebrate collective achievements and learn from group experiences.

• Take the time to acknowledge and celebrate the successes of your collaborative efforts. Recognizing each team member's contributions can build a sense of unity and appreciation.

• Reflect on the experiences of working in a group, both the challenges and the triumphs. Discuss what worked well and what could be improved for future collaborations.

• Use collaborative projects as learning opportunities. Each experience can teach you about teamwork, communication, and the creative process, helping you become a more effective collaborator in the future.

Collaborating with others can significantly enhance creativity and lead to more innovative results. Engaging in collaborative projects, sharing ideas and feedback, and celebrating collective achievements can foster a creative community that supports and inspires everyone involved.

CHAPTER 9

Recap of Key Themes

This book has explored the various aspects of living a fulfilling and happy life through embracing simple pleasures and engaging in creative pursuits. We've delved into topics such as mindfulness, gratitude, the joy of creativity, the importance of connections and community, the benefits of simplicity and decluttering, personal growth, work-life balance, physical and emotional wellness, and the power of nature and collaboration.

• Each chapter has provided actionable steps and detailed sub-chapters to guide you on your journey toward a happier and more content life. By focusing on the present moment, fostering creativity, building meaningful relationships, and prioritizing well-being, you can cultivate a life filled with joy and purpose.

Final Thoughts:

• As you progress, I encourage you to take the actionable steps outlined in this book to heart. Embrace life's simple pleasures, from a beautiful sunset to a heartfelt conversation with a loved one. Engage in creative pursuits that ignite your passion and bring you fulfillment.

• Remember that happiness is a journey, not a destination. It's found in the everyday moments, the connections we make, and the creativity we express. By being mindful, grateful, and intentional in your actions, you can create a life that is not only happy but deeply meaningful.

Invitation for Continued Growth:

• I invite you to continue exploring and implementing the concepts and practices discussed in this book. The journey to happiness and fulfillment is ongoing; there is always more to discover and learn.

• Stay curious, open-minded, and willing to try new things. Seek growth opportunities, whether learning a new skill, connecting with new people, or exploring new ways to express your creativity.

• Remember that you have the power to shape your own happiness. By taking small, consistent steps and embracing the art of happy living, you can create a rich, vibrant, and deeply satisfying life.

This book, "The Art of Happy Living: Simple Pleasures and Creative Pursuits," has provided a comprehensive guide to cultivating a happier and more fulfilled life. I hope it has inspired you to embrace the beauty of simplicity, the joy of creativity, and the power of connection. May your journey be filled with happiness, growth, and endless possibilities.

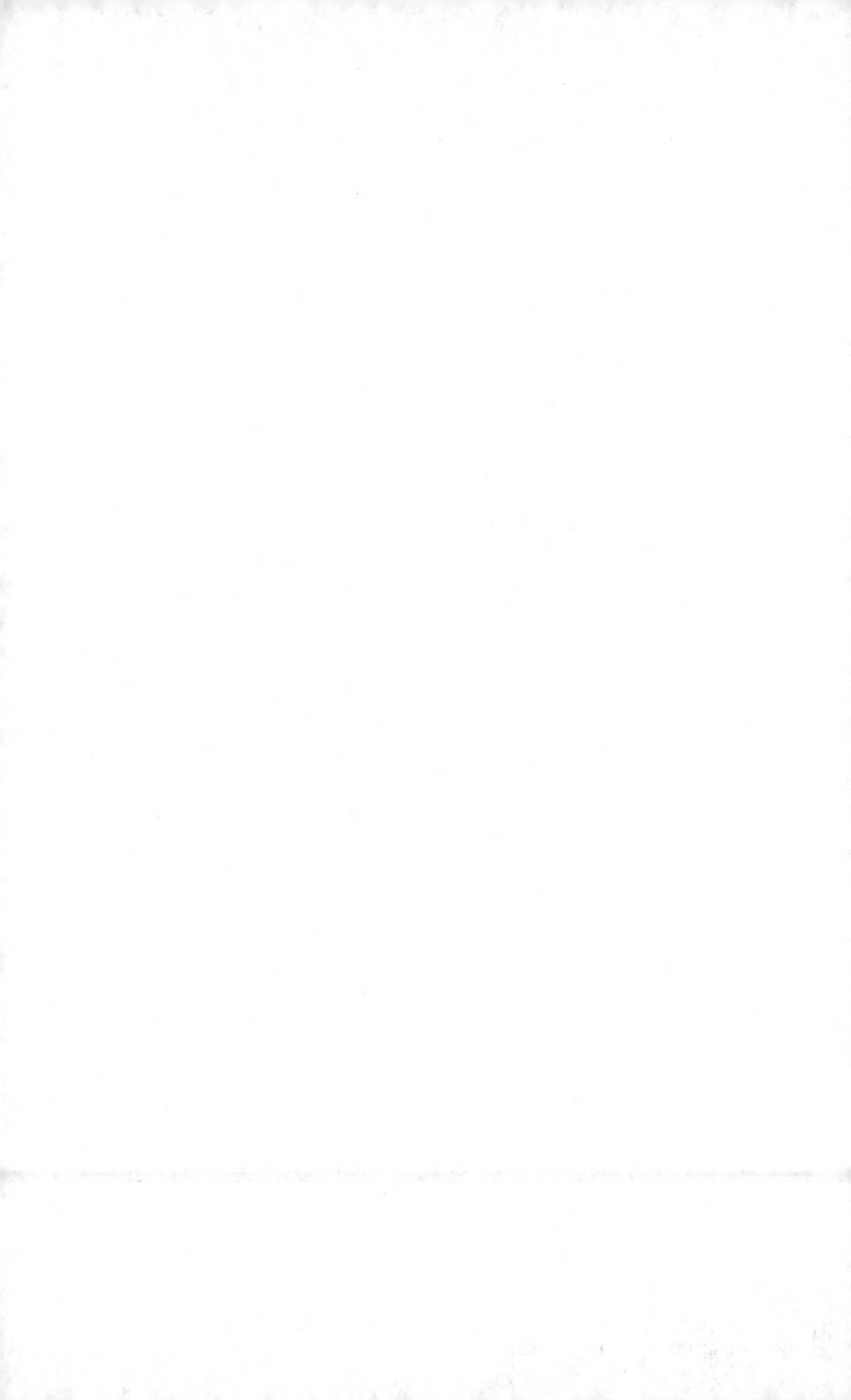